50 Best Paleo Recipes

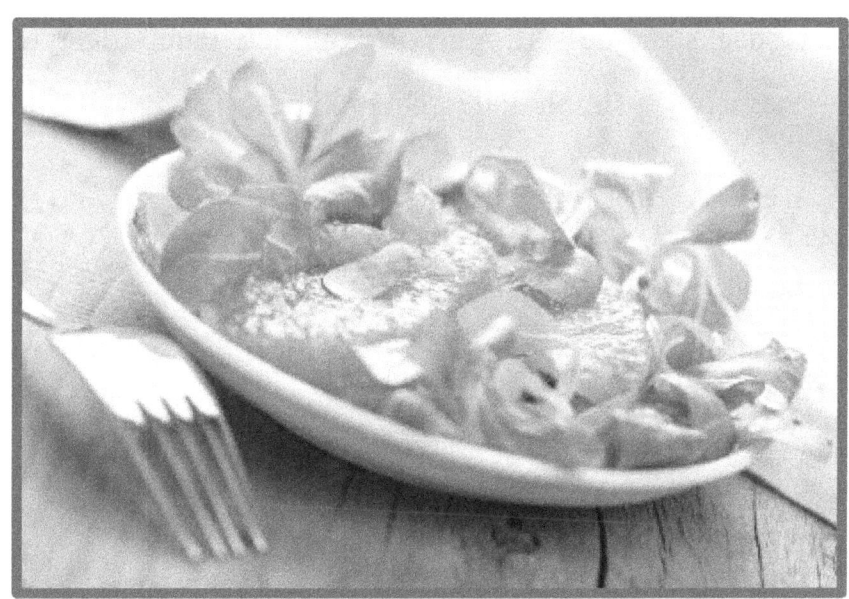

About the Book

If you haven't heard of the Paleo Diet, it is definitely something you should look into. The Paleo Diet is based on the diets of our ancient ancestors and it is the diet that human beings evolved to follow. In this book you will find valuable information about the diet as well as 50 of the best Paleo Diet recipes. Switching to a new diet can be tricky as you figure out all of the rules and guidelines. With the help of this book, however, you will have a wide range of meal options to choose from including breakfast, lunch, dinner, snacks and dessert. Start off your new Paleo lifestyle right by trying out these tasty yet simple Paleo Diet recipes!

Introduction

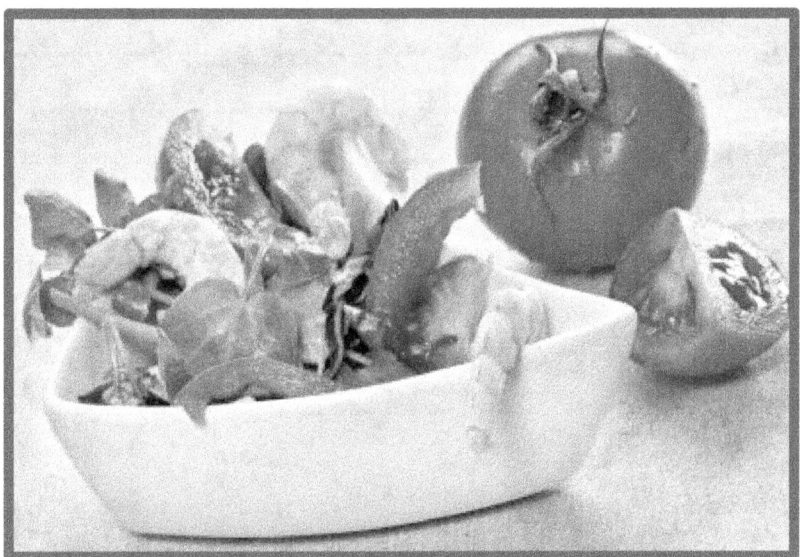

There always seems to be a new fad diet sweeping the health and fitness industry and, with all the diets out there, it may be hard to decide which is the right one for you. The Paleo Diet is more than just a fad diet – it is a healthy lifestyle that provides a number of important health benefits. In addition to ridding your bodies of the toxins found in processed foods, the Paleo Diet is also low in both sodium and sugar. These features, added to the fact that the Paleo Diet is based on whole and nutritious foods, contributes to improved overall health and a decreased risk for chronic disease in followers of the diet.

When you first look into the Paleo Diet you may be tempted to think that it is incredibly restrictive – not only can you no longer eat processed foods but you must also stay away from sugar, grains and dairy products. It is important to remember, however, that the Paleo Diet is more than just a diet. The Paleo Diet is a way of life and, if you are willing to dedicate yourself to it, you are likely to experience a number of significant benefits including improved energy, healthy weight loss, lowered cholesterol and improved insulin response. This book is full of easy, healthy recipes that conform to the guidelines of the Paleo Diet. If you are looking for a little boost to jumpstart your journey with the Paleo Diet, look no further – these recipes are so delicious and satisfying that you will forget you are on a diet at all!

Contents

Breakfast

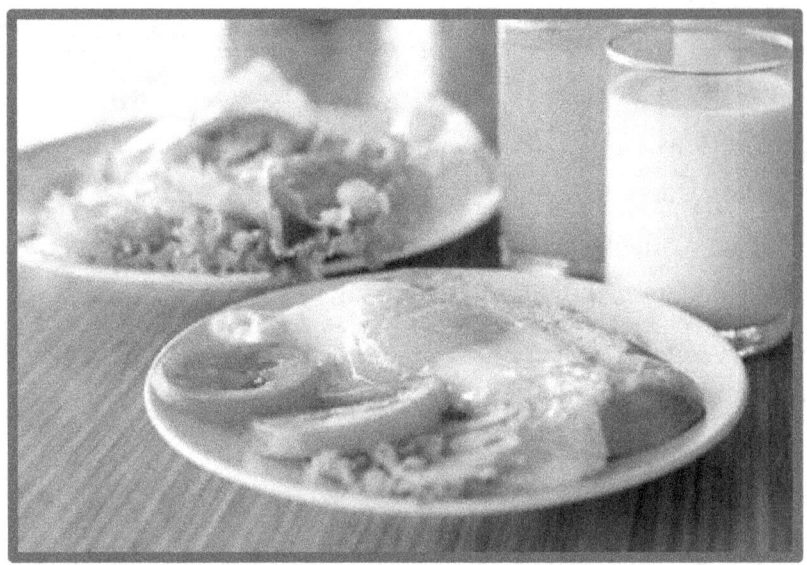

Included in this Section:

Cinnamon Swirled Pancakes

Banana Pecan Muffins

Mushroom and Onion Omelet

Sautéed Sweet Potatoes

Sautéed Tomato Omelet

Zucchini Muffins

Groovy Green Smoothie

Banana Bread

Honey Almond Butter Pancakes

Steak and Eggs

Cinnamon Swirled Pancakes

Prep Time: 15 minutes   **Servings:** 4

Ingredients:

1 cup almond flour
½ cup coconut flour
½ cup unsweetened applesauce
½ cup almond milk
3 eggs, beaten
2 tbsp. raw honey
2 tsp. ground cinnamon
1 tsp. vanilla extract
Coconut oil for cooking

Instructions:

1. Heat a large nonstick skillet over medium heat and grease it with coconut oil.
2. Whisk together the almond flour, coconut flour and ground cinnamon.
3. Beat in the applesauce, almond milk, eggs, honey and vanilla extract. Stir until the batter is smooth.
4. Pour ¼ cup batter into the heated skillet and cook until bubbles form on the surface, about 2 minutes.
5. Flip the pancake and cook until lightly browned on the other side, about 2 minutes. Transfer to a plate and repeat with the remaining ingredients.

Banana Pecan Muffins

Prep Time: 35 minutes **Servings:** 12 to 18

Ingredients:

1 cup almond flour
½ cup coconut flour
3 ripe bananas, mashed
4 large eggs
¼ cup raw honey
¼ cup coconut oil, melted
2 tsp. baking powder
1 tsp. ground cinnamon
½ cup chopped pecans

Instructions:

1. Preheat the oven to 350°F. Line two muffin pans with paper liners and set aside.
2. Whisk together the almond flour, coconut flour, baking powder and ground cinnamon in a bowl.
3. Beat together the eggs, honey and coconut oil. Gradually whisk in the dry ingredients until a smooth batter forms. Fold in the mashed bananas and pecans.
4. Scoop into the prepared muffin pans, filling each cup about 2/3 full.
5. Bake for 20 to 25 minutes until a knife inserted in the center comes out clean.
6. Cool in pans for 10 minutes then turn out onto wire racks to cool completely.

Mushroom and Onion Omelet

Prep Time: 15 minutes   **Servings:** 1

Ingredients:

2 large eggs
1 tsp. coconut oil
1 clove garlic, minced
¼ cup Vidalia onion, diced
¼ cup mushrooms, diced
1 green onion, sliced
½ tsp. salt
¼ tsp. black pepper

Instructions:

1. Beat the eggs together with the garlic, green onion, salt and pepper.
2. Heat the coconut oil in a small nonstick frying pan over medium heat.
3. Pour the eggs into the pan and turn the pan to coat the bottom. Cook for 1 minute.
4. Scrape down the sides of the pan, letting the uncooked egg fill in the empty space.
5. Sprinkle the mushrooms and onion over half the omelet and cook for 2 minutes until the egg is almost set.
6. Fold the empty half of the omelet over the vegetables and cook until set, about 2 more minutes. Transfer to a plate and serve immediately.

Sautéed Sweet Potatoes

Prep Time: 15 minutes   **Servings:** 2

Ingredients:

2 large sweet potatoes, chopped
1 tbsp. coconut oil
1 clove garlic, minced
2 green onions, sliced
1 tsp. salt
½ tsp. black pepper
¼ tsp. paprika

Instructions:

1. Heat the coconut oil in a skillet over medium heat. Add the garlic and cook until fragrant, about 2 minutes.
2. Toss the remaining ingredients in a bowl and add to the skillet.
3. Cook until the sweet potatoes are tender, about 10 minutes. Serve hot.

Sautéed Tomato Basil Omelet

Prep Time: 15 minutes   **Servings:** 1

Ingredients:

2 large eggs
2 tsp. coconut oil, divided
1 clove garlic, minced
1 tomato, chopped
2 fresh basil leaves, chopped
2 tbsp. diced onion
½ tsp. salt
¼ tsp. black pepper

Instructions:

1. Heat 1 tsp. coconut oil in a small skillet over medium heat. Add the garlic and cook until fragrant, about 2 minutes.
2. Stir in the tomato, basil and onion. Cook for about 2 minutes then remove to a small bowl.
3. Beat together the eggs, salt and black pepper.
4. Heat the other tsp. coconut oil in the skillet and pour in the eggs. Cook for 1 minute.
5. Scrape down the sides of the pan, letting the uncooked egg fill in the empty space.
6. Sprinkle the cooked tomato, basil and onion over half the omelet and cook for 2 minutes until the egg is almost set.
7. Fold the empty half of the omelet over the vegetables and cook until set, about 2 more minutes. Transfer to a plate and serve immediately.

Chocolate Zucchini Muffins

Prep Time: **Servings:**

Ingredients:

1 cup almond flour
½ cup coconut flour
1 cup grated zucchini
4 large eggs
¼ cup raw honey
¼ cup coconut oil, melted
2 tbsp. unsweetened cocoa powder
2 tsp. baking powder
½ tsp. ground cinnamon

Instructions:

1. Preheat the oven to 350°F. Line two muffin pans with paper liners and set aside.
2. Whisk together the almond flour, coconut flour, cocoa powder and baking powder in a bowl.
3. Beat together the eggs, honey and coconut oil. Gradually whisk in the dry ingredients until a smooth batter forms. Fold in the grated zucchini.
4. Scoop into the prepared muffin pans, filling each cup about 2/3 full.
5. Bake for 20 to 25 minutes until a knife inserted in the center comes out clean.
6. Cool in pans for 10 minutes then turn out onto wire racks to cool completely.

Groovy Green Smoothie

Prep Time: 5 minutes   **Servings:** 2

Ingredients:

1 cup baby spinach
1 cup fresh kale
1 frozen banana, sliced
½ cup orange juice
½ cup coconut milk
2 tbsp. raw honey
½ cup ice cubes

Instructions:

1. Combine the ingredients in a blender, blending until well combined.
2. Add more ice to thicken, if desired.
3. Divide between two glasses and serve immediately.

Banana Bread

Prep Time: 1 hour 15 minutes   **Servings:** 10

Ingredients:

1 ½ cups almond flour
¼ cups coconut flour
2 ripe bananas, mashed
3 eggs, separated
¼ cup raw honey
¼ cup olive oil
2 tsp. ground cinnamon
1 tsp. baking powder
½ cup chopped walnuts (optional)

Instructions:

1. Preheat the oven to 350° and grease a loaf pan. Set aside.
2. Whisk together the almond flour, coconut flour, ground cinnamon and baking powder in a mixing bowl.
3. Beat the eggs, honey and olive oil in a bowl. Gradually beat in the dry ingredients until a smooth batter forms.
4. Stir in the mashed bananas and the chopped walnuts.
5. Pour the batter into the prepared pan and bake for 1 hour or until the top of the bread is golden brown.
6. Cool slightly before slicing to serve.

Honey Almond Butter Pancakes

Prep Time: **Servings:**

Ingredients:

1 cup almond flour
½ cup coconut flour
½ cup almond butter
½ cup almond milk
3 eggs, beaten
2 tbsp. raw honey
1 tsp. vanilla extract
Coconut oil for cooking

Instructions:

1. Heat a large nonstick skillet over medium heat and grease it with coconut oil.
2. Whisk together the almond flour and coconut flour in a small bowl.
3. Beat in the almond butter, almond milk, eggs, honey and vanilla extract. Stir until the batter is smooth.
4. Pour ¼ cup batter into the heated skillet and cook until bubbles form on the surface, about 2 minutes.
5. Flip the pancake and cook until lightly browned on the other side, about 2 minutes. Transfer to a plate and repeat with the remaining ingredients.

Steak and Eggs

Prep Time: 15 minutes   **Servings:** 2

Ingredients:

½ lbs. sirloin steak, chopped
4 large eggs
2 tbsp. diced onion
2 tsp. coconut oil, divided
Salt and pepper to taste

Instructions:

1. Heat 1 tsp. coconut oil in a small skillet over medium heat. Add the steak and onions, season with salt and pepper to taste.
2. Cook for 3 to 5 minutes until the steak is browned then transfer to a plate.
3. Reheat the skillet with 1 tsp. coconut oil.
4. Crack the eggs into the skillet and cook until done to your liking. Serve with the steak and onions.

Lunch

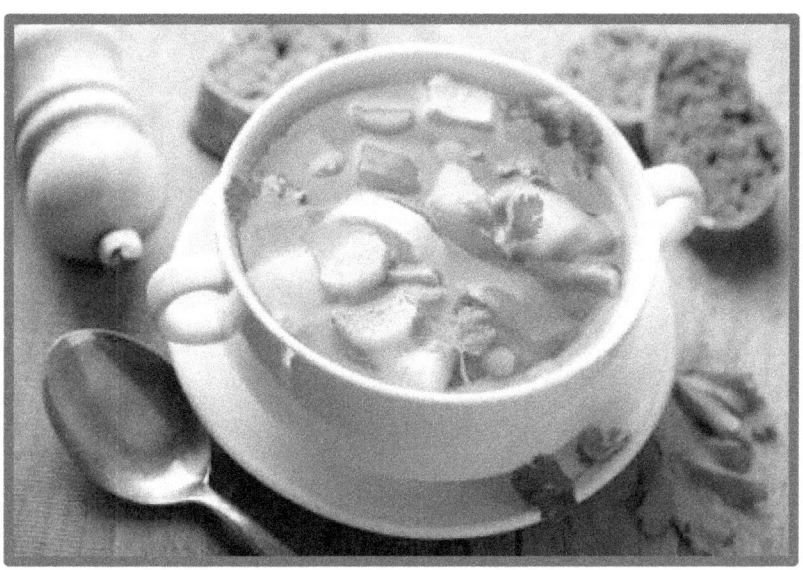

Included in this Section:

Hot Hamburger Casserole

Spicy Chicken Vegetable Soup

Tuna Salad on Lettuce

Raspberry Pecan Salad

Creamy Tomato Bisque

Sweet Potato Stew

Fresh Fruit Salad

Thai Chicken Curry

Grilled Chicken with Veggies

Sweet Sesame Salad

Hot Hamburger Casserole

Prep Time: 35 minutes   **Servings:** 4

Ingredients:

1 lbs. lean ground beef
1 cup onion, chopped
¾ cup almond milk
½ cup almond flour
2 eggs
½ tsp. sea salt
¼ tsp. black pepper

Instructions:

1. Preheat the oven to 400°F. Grease a glass baking dish or pie plate.
2. Heat a skillet over medium heat and add the beef and onions. Cook until the beef is browned and the onions tender. Drain the fat.
3. Transfer the meat and onions to the dish.
4. Whisk together the remaining ingredients and pour into the dish.
5. Bake for 25 to 30 minutes or until a knife inserted in the center comes out clean.
6. Cool slightly before serving.

Spicy Chicken Vegetable Soup

Prep Time: 2 hours   **Servings:** 4

Ingredients:

1 tsp. coconut oil
2 cloves garlic, minced
1 onion, chopped
2 carrots, sliced
2 stalks celery, sliced
1 parsnip, peeled and chopped
¼ cup chopped parsley
1 tsp. dried oregano
1 tsp. sea salt
½ tsp. black pepper
¼ tsp. cayenne pepper
2 cups cooked chicken, chopped
6 cups chicken stock

Instructions:

1. Heat the coconut oil in a stockpot over medium heat. Add the garlic and cook until fragrant, about 2 minutes.
2. Add the onion, carrots, celery and parsnip. Cook for 10 minutes.
3. Stir in the remaining ingredients and bring to a boil.
4. Reduce heat and simmer, covered, for 1 ½ hours. Serve hot.

Tuna Salad on Lettuce

Prep Time: 10 minutes   **Servings:** 2

Ingredients:
5 cups chopped romaine lettuce
2 cans tuna, drained
2 hardboiled eggs, peeled
1 large stalk celery, diced
2 tbsp. olive oil
2 tbsp. minced red onion
1 tbsp. white wine vinegar
½ tsp. sea salt
¼ tsp. black pepper

Instructions:

1. Divide the romaine between two plates. Dice the eggs.
2. Shred the tuna in a bowl and add the eggs, celery and onion. Stir to combine.
3. Stir in the remaining ingredients until well combined.
4. Serve on top of the lettuce.

Raspberry Pecan Salad

Prep Time: 10 minutes   **Servings:** 2

Ingredients:

4 cups baby spinach
2 cups chopped romaine
2 green onions, sliced
½ cup mushrooms, sliced
¼ cup red onion, sliced
1 ¼ cup raspberries, divided
2 tbsp. olive oil
1 tsp. apple cider vinegar
½ cup chopped pecans

Instructions:

1. Combine the spinach, romaine, green onions, mushrooms and red onion in a large bowl. Toss to combine then divide between two plates.
2. Pulse ¼ cup raspberries in a food processor until blended. Pulse in the olive oil and apple cider vinegar.
3. Top the salads with the chopped pecans and remaining raspberries.
4. Drizzle with dressing and serve immediately.

Creamy Tomato Bisque

Prep Time: 1 hour   **Servings:** 4

Ingredients:

2 lbs. tomatoes, halved
1 onion, chopped
1 tbsp. coconut oil
2 cloves garlic, minced
1 cup vegetable broth
½ cup canned coconut milk
1 tsp. dried oregano
1 tsp. dried basil
½ tsp. black pepper

Instructions:

1. Heat the coconut oil in a stockpot and add the garlic. Cook until fragrant, about 2 minutes.
2. Stir in the onion and tomatoes and cook until the tomatoes are tender, about 10 minutes or so.
3. Stir in the vegetable broth and bring to a boil. Reduce heat and simmer, covered, for 30 minutes.
4. Puree the soup with an immersion blender until smooth. Whisk in the milk and spices. Simmer for 5 minutes before serving.

Sweet Potato Stew

Prep Time: 15 minutes   **Servings:** 6

Ingredients:

2 lbs. sweet potatoes, chopped
1 tbsp. coconut oil
2 cloves garlic, minced
2 carrots, sliced
2 stalks celery, sliced
1 onion, chopped
2 cups vegetable broth
1 tsp. dried oregano
½ tsp. sea salt
¼ tsp. pepper

Instructions:

1. Heat the coconut oil in a skillet on medium heat. Add the garlic and cook until fragrant, about two minutes.
2. Add the sweet potatoes and cook until lightly browned, about 5 minutes.
3. Combine the sweet potatoes and the remaining ingredients in a slow cooker, stirring until well combined.
4. Cover and cook on low heat for 4 to 6 hours. Serve hot.

Fresh Fruit Salad

Prep Time: 5 minutes   **Servings:** 4

Ingredients:

1 mango, pitted and chopped
1 kiwi, peeled and sliced
1 apple, chopped
1 cup chopped cantaloupe
1 cup sliced strawberries
1 cup grapes, halved
¾ tsp. ground cinnamon
¼ tsp. ground nutmeg

Instructions:

1. Combine all the ingredients in a bowl, tossing with the spices.
2. Divide into bowls, serve cold.

Thai Chicken Curry
Prep Time: 1 hour   **Servings:** 4

Ingredients:

1 lbs. boneless chicken, chopped
1 tbsp. coconut oil
2 cloves garlic, minced
1 onion, chopped
1 red pepper, chopped
1 cup chicken stock
1 cup diced tomatoes
1 (14 oz.) can coconut milk
3 tbsp. curry powder
1 tsp. black pepper

Instructions:

1. Heat the coconut oil in a large skillet on medium heat. Add the garlic and cook until fragrant, about two minutes.
2. Add the chicken and cook until lightly browned, about 5 minutes. Stir in the remaining ingredients except for the coconut milk.
3. Bring to a boil then reduce heat and simmer, cooked, for 25 minutes.
4. Stir in the coconut milk and simmer for an additional 15minutes before serving.

Grilled Chicken with Veggies

Prep Time: 40 minutes   **Servings:** 4

Ingredients:

2 lbs. chicken leg quarters
1 red pepper, sliced
1 green pepper, sliced
1 onion, sliced thick
2 tbsp. olive oil
Sea salt and pepper to taste

Instructions:

1. Cover half the grates with aluminum foil then preheat the grill.
2. Season the chicken with salt and pepper. Toss the vegetables with the olive oil.
3. Lay the chicken on the grates and cook for 12 to 15 minutes on each side until cooked through.
4. Spread the vegetables on the foil and cook for 3 minutes on each side until tender.

Sweet Sesame Salad

Prep Time: 10 minutes   **Servings:** 2

Ingredients:

6 cups mixed greens
¼ cup red onion, sliced
1 carrot, julienned
1 stalk celery, sliced thin
2 tbsp. olive oil
2 tbsp. apple cider vinegar
1 tsp. sesame oil
1 tsp. raw honey
1 tsp. sesame seeds

Instructions:

1. Whisk together the olive oil, vinegar, sesame oil and honey in a small bowl. Set aside.
2. Combine the greens, onion, carrot and celery in a large bowl, tossing to combine.
3. Toss the dressing with the salad and divide between two plates.
4. Sprinkle the sesame seeds on top and serve.

Snacks and Appetizers

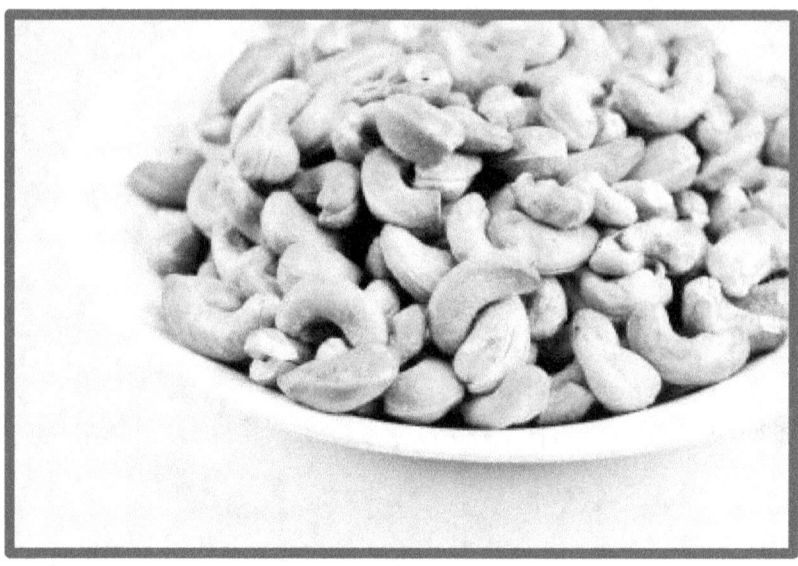

Included in this Section:

Spicy Kale Chips

Strawberry Flaxseed Smoothie

Tasty Trail Mix

Baked Hot Wings

Tropical Fruit Smoothie

Cinnamon Banana Chips

Stuffed Mushrooms

Grilled Veggie Skewers

Shrimp Cocktail

Biscuits with Honey

Spicy Kale Chips

Prep Time: 25 minutes   **Servings:** 2

Ingredients:

1 bunch fresh kale
2 tbsp. olive oil
1 tsp. sea salt
¼ tsp. cayenne pepper

Instructions:

1. Preheat the oven to 350°F. Line a baking sheet with parchment.
2. Break the kale up into pieces and toss with the olive oil, salt and cayenne pepper.
3. Spread the kale chunks on the prepared baking sheet and bake for 15 to 20 minutes until crisp.

Strawberry Flaxseed Smoothie

Prep Time: 5 minutes   **Servings:** 2

Ingredients:

1 ½ cups frozen strawberries
1 banana, sliced
½ cup orange juice
½ cup coconut milk
1 tbsp. raw honey
1 tsp. flaxseed
½ cup ice cubes

Instructions:

1. Combine the ingredients in a blender, blending until well combined.
2. Add more ice to thicken, if desired.
3. Divide between two glasses and serve immediately.

Tasty Trail Mix

Prep Time: 5 minutes   **Servings:** 4

Ingredients:

1 cup raw cashews
½ cup pecan halves
½ cup toasted almonds
½ cup dried cranberries
½ cup dried apricots, chopped
¼ cup raw sunflower seeds
1 tsp. sea salt
¼ tsp. paprika

Instructions:

1. Combine the nuts, dried fruit and sunflower seeds in a bowl.
2. Toss the mixture with the sea salt and paprika.
3. Store in an air-tight container.

Baked Hot Wings

Prep Time: 1 hour   **Servings:** 4

Ingredients:

2 lbs. chicken wings
1 tsp. sea salt
½ tsp. black pepper
¼ tsp. garlic powder
¼ tsp. cayenne pepper
¼ tsp. chili powder

Instructions:

1. Bring a large pot of water to boil and add the chicken wings. Boil for 7 minutes then dry them with a paper towel.
2. Preheat the oven to 450°F. Combine the spices in a small bowl.
3. Spread the wings on a baking sheet and sprinkle the spice mixture over them.
4. Bake for 30 minutes then flip the wings and bake for another 10 minutes.

Tropical Fruit Smoothie

Prep Time: 5 minutes   **Servings:** 2

Ingredients:

2 frozen bananas, sliced
1 mango, peeled and chopped
1 cup frozen pineapple chunks
1 cup orange juice
½ cup coconut milk
1 tbsp. raw honey
½ cup ice cubes

Instructions:

1. Combine the ingredients in a blender, blending until well combined.
2. Add more ice to thicken, if desired.
3. Divide between two glasses and serve immediately.

Cinnamon Banana Chips

Prep Time: 2 hours   **Servings:** 2

Ingredients:

4 bananas, peeled
2 tsp. ground cinnamon

Instructions:

1. Preheat the oven to 200°F. Line a baking sheet with parchment paper.
2. Slice the bananas about 1/8th-inch thick and toss them with the ground cinnamon.
3. Spread the banana slices on the baking dish and bake for 2 to 3 hours until crisp.

Stuffed Mushrooms

Prep Time: **Servings:** 4

Ingredients:

2 lbs. baby portabella mushrooms
2 tbsp. olive oil
½ lbs. raw shrimp
¼ cup red onions, chopped
¼ cup fresh cilantro, chopped
¼ cup diced tomatoes
½ tsp. sea salt
¼ tsp. black pepper

Instructions:

1. Preheat the oven to 450°F.
2. Remove the stems from the mushrooms and set aside.
3. Line a baking sheet with parchment paper and arrange the mushroom caps, upside down, on the sheet. Brush with olive oil.
4. Bake the mushroom caps for 5 to 10 minutes.
5. Combine the remaining ingredients in a food processor and pulse until finely chopped.
6. Spoon about a teaspoon of the shrimp mixture into each mushroom cap and bake for 8 to 10 minutes until the shrimp is cooked through.

Grilled Veggie Skewers
Prep Time: 15 minutes   **Servings:** 4

Ingredients:

1 cup button mushrooms
1 onion, cut into 1-inch chunks
1 green pepper, cut into 1-inch chunks
1 red pepper, cut into 1-inch chunks
2 tbsp. olive oil
1 tsp. sea salt
½ tsp. black pepper
½ tsp. garlic powder
Wooden skewers

Instructions:

1. Soak the skewers in water overnight.
2. Preheat the grill and season the grates with olive oil.
3. Whisk together the olive oil, sea salt, pepper and garlic powder in a small bowl.
4. Combine the vegetables in a bowl and toss with the olive oil mixture.
5. Slide the vegetables onto the wooden skewers and grill for 2 to 3 minutes on each side until charred. Serve hot.

Shrimp Cocktail

Prep Time: 5 minutes   **Servings:** 4

Ingredients:

1 lbs. raw shrimp, peeled and deveined
1 cup tomato sauce
1 tbsp. mustard
2 tsp. horseradish
1 tsp. lemon juice

Instructions:

1. Combine all ingredients except for the shrimp in a bowl, whisking to combine.
2. Serve the shrimp with the sauce.

Biscuits with Honey

Prep Time: 25 minutes   **Servings:** 4

Ingredients:

1 cup almond flour
6 egg whites
¼ cup almond milk
2 tbsp. olive oil
1 tsp. baking soda
¼ tsp. sea salt
Raw honey

Instructions:

1. Preheat the oven to 400°F and line a baking sheet with parchment paper.
2. Beat together the flour, almond milk, olive oil, baking soda and sea salt in a mixing bowl.
3. Beat the egg whites separately until frothy then stir into the batter.
4. Drop the batter in quarter-cup scoops onto the prepared baking sheet. Bake for 15 to 18 minutes until lightly browned. Serve warm.

Dinner

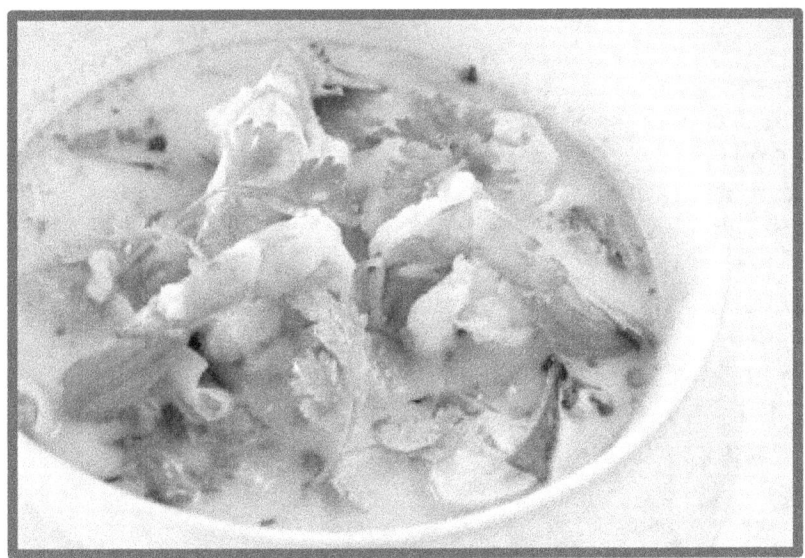

<u>Included in this Section:</u>

Roasted Chicken with Veggies

Tender Beef Pot Roast

Vegetable Shrimp Curry

Pork and Vegetable Stir-Fry

Baked Mango Haddock

Turkey Burgers

Maple Walnut Chicken Thighs

Spicy Lamb Stew

Peppered Flank Steak with Mushrooms

Baked Pork Chops

Roasted Chicken with Veggies

Prep Time: 1 hour   **Servings:** 4

Ingredients:

2 lbs. chicken legs and thighs
1 tbsp. coconut oil
2 cloves garlic, minced
2 sweet potatoes, chopped
2 carrots, sliced
1 cup broccoli florets
1 onion, quartered
¼ cup chicken stock
2 tbsp. olive oil
1 tsp. dried rosemary
1 tsp. dried basil
Sea salt and pepper to taste

Instructions:

1. Preheat the oven to 375°F. Whisk together the chicken stock, olive oil, rosemary and basil. Set aside.
2. Season the chicken with sea salt and pepper to taste.
3. Heat the coconut oil in a large skillet over medium heat. Add the garlic and cook until fragrant, about 2 minutes.
4. Add the chicken and cook until browned, about 3 minutes. Flip and brown on the other side.
5. Transfer the chicken to a glass baking dish and add the vegetables around it.
6. Drizzle the chicken stock mixture over the chicken and vegetables and cook until the chicken is cooked through, about 45 minutes.

Tender Beef Pot Roast

Prep Time: 3 hours   **Servings:** 6

Ingredients:

4 ½ tsp. beef chuck roast
2 tsp. coconut oil
3 cloves garlic, minced
2 carrots, sliced
2 onions, quartered
1 cup button mushrooms
1 cup beef stock
1 tsp. dried rosemary
1 tsp. dried oregano
½ tsp. black pepper

Instructions:

1. Heat the coconut oil in a Dutch oven over medium heat and add the garlic. Cook until fragrant, about 2 minutes.
2. Add the beef and cook until browned on the bottom, about 3 minutes. Turn and cook until browned on the other sides.
3. Combine the vegetables in the Dutch oven around the meat.
4. Whisk together the remaining ingredients and pour over the ingredients in the Dutch oven.
5. Cover and cook on high heat for 2 to 4 hours or until the beef is tender. Shred with two forks and serve with vegetables.

Vegetable Shrimp Curry

Prep Time: 1 hour   **Servings:** 4

Ingredients:

1 lbs. raw shrimp, peeled and deveined
1 tbsp. coconut oil
3 cloves garlic, minced
1 red pepper, chopped
1 green pepper, chopped
1 onion, chopped
1 cup bean sprouts
1 cup vegetable stock
1 cup diced tomatoes
1 (14 oz.) can coconut milk
3 tbsp. curry powder
1 tsp. black pepper

Instructions:

1. Heat the coconut oil in a large skillet on medium heat. Add the garlic and cook until fragrant, about two minutes.
2. Add the vegetables and cook for 5 minutes. Stir in the vegetable stock, tomatoes, curry powder and pepper.
3. Bring to a boil then reduce heat and simmer, cooked, for 25 minutes.
4. Stir in the coconut milk and shrimp then simmer for an additional 15minutes before serving.

Pork and Vegetable Stir-Fry

Prep Time: 35 minutes   **Servings:** 4

Ingredients:

1 lbs. boneless pork loin, sliced
1 cup broccoli florets
1 cup cauliflower florets
2 carrots, sliced
1 red pepper, chopped
1 green pepper, chopped
¼ cup coconut aminos
2 tbsp. orange juice
1 tbsp. honey
1 tsp. dried ginger
2 cloves garlic, minced
Coconut oil for cooking

Instructions:

1. Heat a large skillet over medium heat and season with coconut oil.
2. Add the peppers and cook until tender, about 5 minutes. Transfer the peppers to a bowl and reheat the skillet.
3. Season the skillet with coconut oil and add the broccoli, cauliflower and carrots. Cook for 7 to 10 minutes until tender. Transfer to the bowl.
4. Reheat the skillet and add the pork. Cook until browned, about 5 minutes.
5. Whisk together the remaining ingredients and push the pork to the sides of the skillet. Add the sauce and cook until bubbly, about 2 minutes.
6. Stir in the pork and vegetables and cook until heated through, about 3 minutes.

Baked Mango Haddock

Prep Time: 20 minutes   **Servings:** 4

Ingredients:

2 lbs. haddock fillet
2 tbsp. olive oil
1 tbsp. lemon juice
½ tsp. black pepper
¼ tsp. garlic powder
1 mango, peeled and chopped
1 tbsp. minced red onion
1 tbsp. chopped cilantro

Instructions:

1. Preheat the oven to 350°F. Lightly grease a roasting pan.
2. Whisk together the olive oil and lemon juice and brush over the fillets. Season with pepper and garlic powder.
3. Bake for 12 to 15 minutes until the flesh flakes easily with a fork.
4. Combine the mango, red onion and cilantro in a bowl. Serve with the fish.

Turkey Burgers

Prep Time: 20 minutes   **Servings:** 4

Ingredients:

1 ½ lbs. lean ground turkey
2 tbsp. almond flour
2 tbsp. onion, minced
2 tbsp. fresh cilantro, chopped
1 egg, beaten
½ tsp. sea salt
½ tsp. black pepper
¼ tsp. chili powder

Instructions:

1. Preheat the broiler on your oven and lightly grease a roasting pan.
2. Combine all ingredients except the egg and turkey in a bowl, stirring to combine.
3. Mix in the turkey by hand then mix in the beaten egg.
4. Shape the turkey mixture into patties and place on the roasting pan.
5. Broil for 3 to 5 minutes on each side until cooked through.

Maple Walnut Chicken Thighs

Prep Time: 1 hour   **Servings:** 4

Ingredients:

2 lbs. bone-in chicken thighs
1 tbsp. coconut oil
¼ cup maple syrup
1 tsp. walnut oil
½ cup pecans
Sea salt and pepper to taste

Instructions:

1. Pulse the pecans in a food processor until finely chopped.
2. Heat the coconut oil in a large skillet over medium heat.
3. Season the chicken with salt and pepper and add to the skillet. Cook until lightly browned, about 3 minutes. Flip and cook until browned on the other side.
4. Preheat the oven to 350°F.
5. Transfer the chicken to a glass baking dish.
6. Drizzle the maple syrup over the chicken and sprinkle with chopped pecans.
7. Bake for 45 minutes or until the chicken is cooked through. Serve hot.

Spicy Lamb Stew

Prep Time: 1 ½ hours   **Servings:** 6

Ingredients:

3 ½ lbs. boneless lamb, chopped
2 tbsp. coconut oil
3 cloves garlic, minced
2 cups cabbage, sliced
1 parsnip, peeled and chopped
1 onion, quartered
2 carrots, sliced
2 stalks celery, sliced
1 cup beef broth
1 tsp. dried marjoram
1 tsp. dried basil
½ tsp. black pepper
½ tsp. cayenne pepper

Instructions:

1. Whisk together the broth and spices. Set aside.
2. Heat the coconut oil in a Dutch oven over medium heat and add the garlic. Cook until fragrant, about 2 minutes.
3. Add the lamb and cook until browned, about 5 minutes.
4. Stir in the parsnip, onion, carrots and celery. Cook for 10 minutes until tender.
5. Pour the broth mixture into the Dutch oven then reduce heat and simmer for 30 minutes.
6. Stir in the cabbage and simmer for an additional 30 minutes before serving.

Peppered Flank Steak with Mushrooms

Prep Time: 25 minutes   **Servings:** 4

Ingredients:

2 lbs. flank steak
1 lbs. mushrooms, sliced
1 tbsp. coconut oil
2 cloves garlic, minced
2 tsp. fresh ground pepper

Instructions:

1. Preheat the broiler in your oven and lightly grease a roasting pan.
2. Season the steak with pepper and place on the roasting pan.
3. Broil the steak for 2 to 3 minutes on each side until cooked to the desired temperature.
4. Heat the coconut oil in a skillet over medium heat. Add the garlic and cook until fragrant, about 2 minutes.
5. Add the mushrooms and cook until browned, about 5 minutes.
6. Serve the steak with the sautéed mushrooms on top.

Baked Pork Chops

Prep Time: 30 minutes   **Servings:** 4

Ingredients:

2 lbs. bone-in pork chops
1 tbsp. olive oil
¾ tsp. sea salt
½ tsp. black pepper
½ tsp. dried rosemary

Instructions:

1. Preheat the oven to 400°F. Lightly grease a roasting pan.
2. Brush the chops with olive oil and season with the salt, pepper and rosemary. Place the chops on the baking sheet.
3. Bake for 25 to 30 minutes or until cooked through. Serve hot.

Dessert

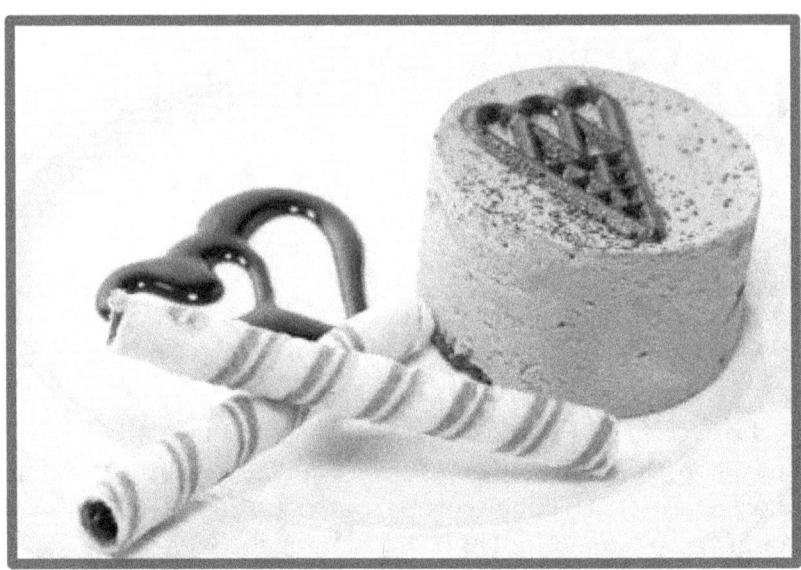

Included in this Section:

Mixed Berry Sorbet

Cherry Chocolate Mousse

Chocolate Chip Cookies

Fresh Fruit Popsicles

Double Chocolate Brownies

Hot Apple Crisp

Lemon Blueberry Cupcakes

Easy Baked Apples

Chocolate-Dipped Fruit

Strawberry Banana Crepes

Mixed Berry Sorbet
Prep Time: 14 minutes   **Servings:** 4

Ingredients:

1 cup sliced strawberries
1 cup fresh blueberries
1 cup fresh raspberries
1 ½ cups water
½ cup raw honey
2 tbsp. lemon juice
½ tsp. lemon zest

Instructions:

1. Combine the water and honey in a small saucepan and cook until the honey is melted.
2. Add the berries and bring the mixture to a boil. Reduce heat and simmer until the berries are soft, stirring occasionally.
3. Strain the berry mixture into a bowl through a sieve and stir in the lemon juice and lemon zest.
4. Cover the bowl and chill for 3 hours until cold.
5. Transfer the liquid to an ice cream maker and freeze according to the manufacturer's instructions. Serve cold.

Cherry Chocolate Mousse

Prep Time: 15 minutes   **Servings:** 4

Ingredients:

2 cups coconut milk
1 avocado, pitted
¼ cup pitted cherries
¼ cup raw honey
1 tbsp. cocoa powder
1 tsp. vanilla extract

Instructions:

1. Pulse the cherries in a food processor until finely chopped.
2. Add the coconut milk, honey and vanilla extract. Blend until smooth then transfer to a bowl.
3. Whisk in the avocado and cocoa powder until well combined.
4. Divide into dessert cups and chill before serving.

Chocolate Chip Cookies

Prep Time: 35 minutes   **Servings:** 2 dozen

Ingredients:

2 ½ cups almond flour
¼ cup coconut flour
½ cup raw honey
½ cup coconut oil, melted
3 large eggs
2 tbsp. almond milk
1 ½ tsp. baking soda
1 tsp. sea salt
1 tsp. vanilla extract
1 cup mini chocolate chips

Instructions:

1. Preheat oven to 375°F. Line a baking sheet with parchment paper and set aside.
2. Combine the almond flour, coconut flour, baking soda and salt in a bowl.
3. Beat the eggs and honey together on medium speed. Beat in the almond milk and vanilla extract.
4. Gradually add the wet ingredients to the dry, mixing as you pour. Stir in the melted coconut oil.
5. Fold in the chocolate chips.
6. Drop the cookie dough in tablespoon-sized balls onto the prepared cookie sheet, spacing them 2 inches apart.
7. Bake for 8 to 10 minutes or until the edges are browned.

Fresh Fruit Popsicles
Prep Time: 10 minutes   **Servings:** 4

Ingredients:

1 cup fresh strawberries
1 cup blueberries
1 cup raspberries
2 cups water
2 tbsp. raw honey

Instructions:

1. Combine the water and honey in a small saucepan and heat until the honey is melted.
2. Pulse the fruit in a food processor until smooth then add to the saucepan and cook until steaming.
3. Remove from heat and cool to room temperature.
4. Pour the fruit mixture into small paper cups and place a wooden stick in each cup. Freeze until solid.

Chewy Chocolate Brownies
Prep Time: 35 minutes   **Servings:** 12

Ingredients:

2 cups almond flour
¼ cup coconut flour
3 large eggs
¾ cups raw honey
½ cups unsweetened cocoa powder
¼ cup coconut oil, melted
2 tbsp. almond milk
1 tsp. vanilla extract

Instructions:

1. Preheat the oven to 350°F and lightly grease a square 8x8-inch baking dish.
2. Whisk together the honey and melted coconut oil until smooth and combined – warm slightly in the microwave if needed.
3. Combine the almond flour, coconut flour and cocoa powder in a bowl.
4. Transfer the honey mixture to a separate bowl and beat in the eggs and vanilla extract.
5. Gradually beat in the dry ingredients, scraping down the sides of the bowl as needed. Pour into the prepared baking dish.
6. Bake for 20 to 25 minutes until a knife inserted in the center comes out clean.

Hot Apple Crisp

Prep Time: 1 hour 15 minutes   **Servings:** 6

Ingredients:

1 ½ cups pecans
1 tbsp. almond flour
1 large egg, beaten
4 to 5 apples, cored and sliced
1 tbsp. tapioca starch
1 tbsp. raw honey
1 tbsp. lemon juice
1 ½ tsp. ground cinnamon
½ tsp. ground nutmeg

Instructions:

1. Preheat the oven to 350°F and lightly grease a square 8x8-inch baking dish.
2. Pulse the pecans in a food processor until finely chopped then blend in the almond flour and egg. Pulse until smooth and combined.
3. Press the pecan mixture into the prepared baking dish.
4. Combing the remaining ingredients in a bowl and toss to combine. Pour the apple mixture into the baking dish.
5. Bake for 45 minutes to an hour or until the apples are tender and hot.

Lemon Blueberry Cupcakes

Prep Time: 35 minutes   **Servings:** 24

Ingredients:

1 ½ cups almond flour
¼ cup coconut flour
4 eggs plus 2 whites
1 cup almond milk
½ cup raw honey
2 tbsp. lemon juice
1 ½ tsp. baking powder
1 tsp. vanilla extract
1 tsp. lemon zest
1 cup fresh blueberries

Instructions:

1. Preheat the oven to 350°F. Line two muffin pans with paper liners and set aside.
2. Whisk together the almond flour, coconut flour and baking powder in a small bowl. Set aside.
3. Beat the eggs, egg whites, almond milk, honey, lemon juice, vanilla extract and lemon zest in a mixing bowl until well combined.
4. Add the dry ingredients and stir until a smooth batter forms. Fold in the blueberries.
5. Spoon the batter into the prepared pans, filling each cup about 2/3 full.
6. Bake for 25 to 30 minutes until a knife inserted in the center comes out clean.

Easy Baked Apples

Prep Time: 25 minutes   **Servings:** 6

Ingredients:

6 apples, cored
1/3 cup ghee
¼ cup raisins
2 tbsp. chopped walnuts
3 tbsp. raw honey
2 tsp. ground cinnamon

Instructions:

1. Preheat the oven to 350°F. Lightly grease a large glass baking dish.
2. Arrange the apples in the dish.
3. Combine the ghee, raisins, walnuts and cinnamon in a small bowl. Spoon the mixture into the apples.
4. Drizzle the honey over the apples and bake for 15 to 18 minutes or until the apples are tender and hot.

Chocolate-Dipped Fruit

Prep Time: 15 minutes   **Servings:** 4

Ingredients:

2 bananas, peeled and quartered
1 pint fresh strawberries
1 cup semisweet chocolate chips
1 tsp. coconut oil

Instructions:

1. Place the chocolate chips in a heatproof bowl and microwave until melted. Stir in the coconut oil until smooth.
2. Line a baking sheet with parchment paper.
3. Dip the fruit in the chocolate and lay on the baking sheet.
4. Refrigerate for 10 minutes or until the chocolate is hardened.

Strawberry Banana Crepes

Prep Time: 30 minutes   **Servings:** 4

Ingredients:

2 cups full-fat coconut milk
1 ½ cups tapioca flour
½ cup sweet rice flour
2 large eggs, beaten
1 tsp. vanilla or almond extract
1 cup strawberries, sliced
1-2 bananas, sliced
2 tbsp. raw honey

Instructions:

1. Blend the first five ingredients in a mixing bowl, whisking until well combined.
2. Combine the strawberries, banana and honey in a small saucepan over low heat.
3. Heat a medium nonstick skillet over medium heat and scoop about ¼ to 1/3 cup of the batter into it. Turn the pan to evenly coat the bottom.
4. Cook for 2 to 3 minutes until lightly browned.
5. Transfer to a plate and repeat with the remaining batter.
6. Remove the fruit mixture from heat and spoon into the hot crepes, folding them over the fruit.